PREGNANCY GUIDE FOR DADS

WEEK-BY-WEEK COMPLETE CHILDBIRTH GUIDE FOR FIRST TIME DADS AND MOMS

Dora Harris

TABLE OF CONTENTS

INTRODUCTION

6

CHAPTER ONE   11

PREPARATION

11

CHAPTER TWO   18

LIST FOR EXPECTANT MOTHER

18

CHAPTER THREE   25

BASIC THINGS ABOUT PREGNANCY

25

CHAPTER FOUR   32

ROLES OF DAD TO BE

32

CHAPTER FIVE   36

CHALLENGES OF PREGNANCY

36

CHAPTER SIX   43

IMPORTANCE OF PRENATAL VISITS

43

CHAPTER SEVEN   50

SEX DURING PREGNANCY   50

Benefits of Sex During Pregnancy

53

CHAPTER EIGHT   57

MORNING SICKNESS, PREGNANCY BRAIN

AND CRAVING

57

CHAPTER NINE   61
EXPECTATIONS FOR A MODERN DAD

61

CHAPTER TEN   **68**
MAINTAINING HEALTH AND WELLNESS

68

CHAPTER ELEVEN   74
BODY CHANGES

74

CHAPTER TWELVE   **79**
FIRST TRIMESTER

79

CHAPTER THIRTEEN   **84**
BABY AT FIRST TRIMESTER

84

CHAPTER FOURTEEN   88
MOTHER AT FIRST TRIMESTER

88

CHAPTER FIFTEEN   93
A MUST-KNOW-FOR NEW MOMS

93

CHAPTER SIXTEEN   **97**
SECOND   TRIMESTER   AND   ITS
CHALLENGES

98

CHAPTER SEVENTEEN   **104**
DO THIS IN SECOND TRIMESTER

104

CHAPTER EIGHTEEN 108
DEALING WITH WEIGHT LOSS AND WEIGHT GAIN

108

CHAPTER NINETEEN 112
UNTOLD SECRETS 112
    Fetal Development 113
    Appearance 114
    Sensory Development 114
    Reproductive System

114

CHAPTER TWENTY **117**
    HORMONAL SHIFT

117

CHAPTER TWENTY-ONE 121
NEW MOM AND DAD 121
    Parenting Roles and Responsibilities

125

CHAPTER TWENTY-TWO **126**
    THIRD TRIMESTER OVERVIEW 126
    GETTING PASS THIRD TRIMESTER

130

CHAPTER TWENTY-FOUR **135**
    BABY AT THIRD TRIMESTER

135

CHAPTER TWENTY-FIVE 139
CHILDBIRTH 139
    1. Early Labor 139
    2. Active Labor 140
    3. Delivery 141

4. Placental Stage   141
5. Postpartum Period   142
Medical Interventions

142

CHAPTER TWENTY-SIX   143
WHO NAMES THE CHILD ?

144

CHAPTER TWENTY-SEVEN   144
POSTPARTUM JOURNEY   146
Physical Recovery   146
Hormonal Changes   147
Sleep Deprivation   148
Adjusting to Parenthood   149
Postpartum Care   149
After Child's Birth

151

CHAPTER TWENTY-EIGHT   155
BATHING AN INFANT

155

CHAPTER TWENTY-NINE

160

CONCLUSION

160

Esteem Reader   164

INTRODUCTION

In the quiet hush of anticipation, a couple embarks on the transformative odyssey of parenthood. As the positive test strip announces the impending arrival, the heartbeat of excitement quickens. This isn't just a journey for moms alone – it's a voyage for dads, too. Welcome to the "Pregnancy Guide for Dads," a compass through the labyrinth of joy, challenges, and boundless love.

In the initial weeks, the pregnancy is a guarded secret, whispered between partners like a shared dream. Nausea dances with excitement, and the emotional roller coaster begins. Dads, stand by as morning sickness makes its cameo, and the reality of fatherhood flickers into focus. This trimester is about gentle support, understanding cravings, and sharing the joyous secret while navigating the uncharted waters of parenting.

With the first trimester's whispers fading, the second trimester unveils the magic of ultrasound. Dads, witness the fluttering heartbeat, and let the connection deepen. As the baby kicks and tumbles, your role evolves. Dive into the emotional currents of nursery planning, name debates, and shared dreams for the future. This trimester is the bridge between anticipation and palpable reality.

As the due date looms, the third trimester is a symphony of anticipation and preparation. Dads feel the weight of responsibility mingled with joy. Support becomes more tangible – assembling cribs, packing hospital bags, and sharing the glow of excitement. The emotional crescendo of impending fatherhood crescendos, echoing in the last-minute nerves and blissful expectancy.

For every emotion, question, and unexpected twist, "Pregnancy Guide for Dads" is the lantern in the parental adventure. This book weaves practical advice with heartfelt stories, ensuring both moms and dads navigate the twists and turns of pregnancy and parenthood with confidence.

Embark on this emotional roller coaster with "Pregnancy Guide for Dads" – order your copy today and embrace the extraordinary journey to parenthood. Every page is a guide, every story a revelation. Parenthood awaits, and your guidebook is just a click away.

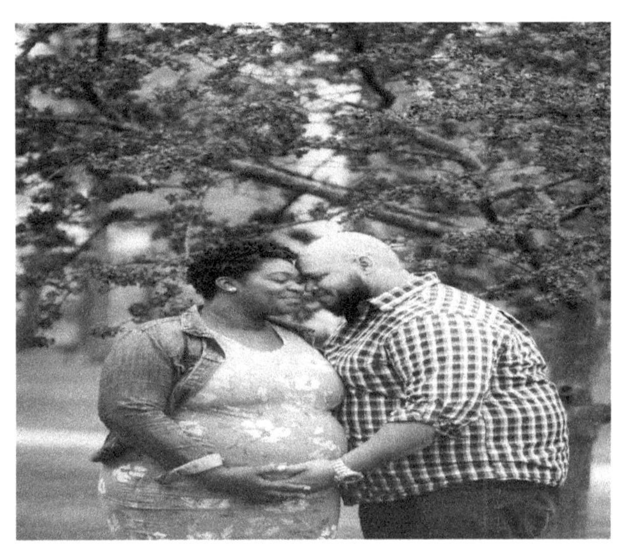

CHAPTER ONE

PREPARATION

Emotional planning and preparation during pregnancy are essential components of ensuring a healthy and positive experience for both the expectant mother and her partner.

Pregnancy brings about a multitude of physical changes, but it also triggers a range of emotions that can vary widely from joy and excitement to anxiety and fear. Here are some key aspects of emotional planning and preparation during pregnancy.

Open Communication:Establishing open and honest communication between partners is very essential. Discussing expectations, concerns, and fears helps build a support system and fosters understanding.

Encourage regular conversations about the emotional journey of pregnancy, addressing both the highs and lows. This helps in identifying any potential emotional challenges early on.

Educational Empowerment: Knowledge is empowering. Attending prenatal classes or reading books on pregnancy and childbirth can help expectant parents understand the physical and emotional changes that occur.Being informed about the stages of pregnancy, potential complications, and the birthing process can alleviate anxiety and promote a sense of control.

Emotional Health Check:Regularly assessing and addressing emotional well-being is crucial. Pregnancy can bring about mood swings and emotional vulnerability.Seek support from friends, colleagues, family, or professionals when need be. Mental health is an integral part of a healthy pregnancy.

Bonding Activities:Engaging in activities that promote bonding between partners and

the growing family is essential. This can include attending prenatal classes together, reading parenting books, or even creating a baby registry as a team.
Establishing a strong emotional connection during pregnancy lays the foundation for a supportive and united parenting approach.

Self-Care Practices:Encourage the practice of self-care to manage stress and nurture emotional well-being. This could include activities such as meditation, gentle exercise, or simply taking time to relax and unwind.Understanding personal needs and prioritizing self-care helps in maintaining emotional balance.

Realistic Expectations:Setting realistic expectations about the changes pregnancy brings is vital. Understanding that both physical and emotional fluctuations are normal can prevent unnecessary stress.Discuss roles and responsibilities as parents, and be open to adjusting expectations as needed.

Prepare for Change:Anticipate and discuss lifestyle changes that may accompany parenthood. This includes adjustments in daily routines, sleep patterns, and social activities.Preparing for these changes together can enhance emotional readiness and create a sense of shared responsibility.

Professional Support:Seeking guidance from healthcare professionals, such as obstetricians, midwives, or counselors, can provide valuable insights and support. Attend prenatal appointments together to stay informed about the progress of the pregnancy and address any concerns as a team.

Emotional planning and preparation during pregnancy involve proactive communication, mutual support, education, and self-care.

By approaching pregnancy as a shared emotional journey, expectant parents can

build a strong foundation for a positive and
healthy transition to parenthood.

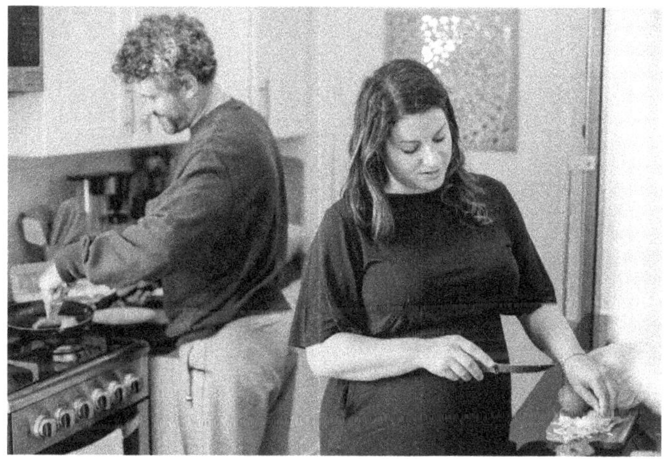

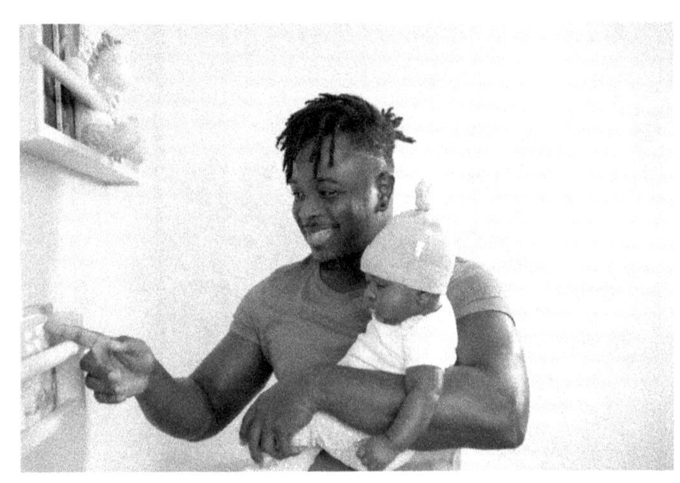

CHAPTER TWO

LIST FOR EXPECTANT MOTHER

Preparing for the arrival of a new baby is an exciting and essential part of pregnancy. An expectant mother needs to ensure that she has all the necessary items to provide a safe and comfortable environment for her newborn. Here is a comprehensive list of things an expectant mother should consider buying.

Maternity Clothing: As the baby bump grows, comfortable and stretchy maternity clothes become essential. This includes maternity jeans, tops, dresses, and sleepwear designed to accommodate a changing body.

Prenatal Vitamins: Essential for the health of both mother and baby, prenatal vitamins provide necessary nutrients like folic acid, iron, and calcium that may be lacking in a regular diet.

Nursery Furniture: Prepare the baby's nursery with a crib, changing table, and a comfortable chair for breastfeeding or bonding moments.

Baby Clothes: Stock up on newborn and 0-3 months baby clothes, including onesies, sleepers, hats, and socks.
Diapers and Wipes: A significant part of early parenthood involves diaper changes. Stock up on both disposable and/or cloth diapers, along with baby wipes.

Feeding Essentials: Whether breastfeeding or using formula, a mother needs nursing bras, breast pads, bottles, and a breast pump if planning to express milk.

Maternity Underwear: Comfortable and supportive underwear designed for pregnancy can make a significant difference.

Pregnancy Pillow: A full-body pillow can provide support for better sleep and alleviate discomfort during pregnancy.

Car Seat: A car seat is mandatory for hospital trips and other outings. Install it well before the due date and ensure it meets safety standards.

Stroller: A stroller is a must-have for easy transportation of the baby. Choose one that suits your lifestyle, whether it's a lightweight stroller for city living or a jogging stroller for active parents.

Baby Carrier: For hands-free mobility and bonding, a baby carrier or sling is invaluable.

Swaddle Blankets: Swaddling helps soothe newborns and promotes better sleep.

Baby Bathtub: Make bath time safe and enjoyable with a baby bathtub that is appropriately sized and equipped with a non-slip surface.

Diaper Bag: An organized and spacious diaper bag is essential for carrying baby essentials when on the go.

Breastfeeding Pillow: A comfortable nursing pillow can make breastfeeding more relaxed for both mother and baby.

Baby Clothes Detergent: Use a mild, baby-safe detergent to wash the baby's clothes, blankets, and other fabric items.

Health and Safety Items: Include items such as a baby thermometer, baby nail clippers, and a first aid kit for minor injuries.

Baby Monitor: A baby monitor provides peace of mind by allowing parents to keep an eye on the baby while they are in another room.

Changing Pad: A portable changing pad is handy for on-the-go diaper changes.

Mom-to-Be Pampering Items: Treat the expectant mother with self-care items such as maternity skincare products, comfortable slippers, and a cozy robe.

By preparing in advance and acquiring these essential items, an expectant mother can ensure a smoother transition into parenthood, focusing on the joy and bonding moments with the new addition to the family.

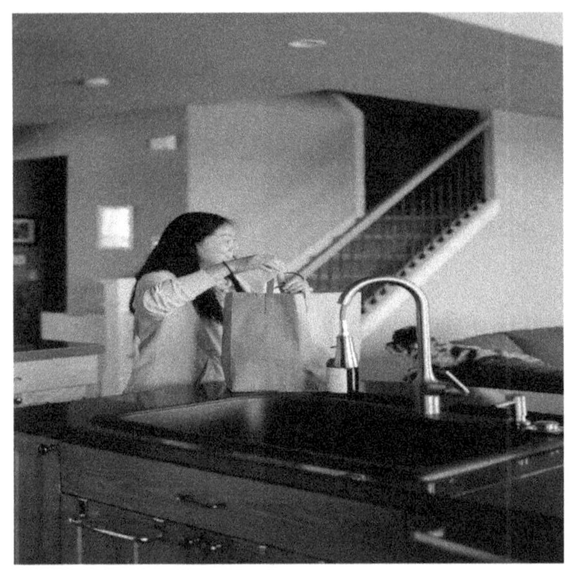

CHAPTER THREE

BASIC THINGS ABOUT PREGNANCY

Pregnancy is a great and transformative journey that marks the beginning of a new phase of life. This incredible process involves the fusion of an egg and sperm, leading to the formation of a zygote that eventually develops into a complex organism within the mother's womb.

Understanding the basics of pregnancy is crucial for expectant parents to navigate this period with care and knowledge. Conception typically occurs during the woman's menstrual cycle, with the release of an egg from the ovaries. This egg then travels through the fallopian tubes, where fertilization by sperm may take place.

Once fertilized, the zygote begins its journey towards the uterus, where it implants itself into the uterine lining. This marks the official beginning of pregnancy. Pregnancy is divided into three trimesters, each lasting about three months. The first trimester is a crucial period of organ formation and rapid development.

The mother may experience symptoms such as morning sickness, fatigue, and breast tenderness during this time. It is also when the baby's heartbeat becomes detectable, and vital organs like the brain and spine begin to take shape.

The second trimester is often considered the most comfortable for many women. Morning sickness tends to subside, and the baby's movements become noticeable. This trimester is characterized by significant growth as the baby's bones harden, and organs continue to mature.

Around the midpoint of pregnancy, an ultrasound can reveal the baby's gender.

The third trimester brings the final stages of development, with the baby's organs reaching full maturity. The mother may experience increased discomfort due to the growing size of the baby and pressure on internal organs. Regular check-ups become essential, monitoring both the mother's and baby's health.

Maintaining a healthy lifestyle is crucial throughout pregnancy. A balanced diet that includes essential nutrients like folic acid, iron, and calcium is vital for the baby's growth. Regular, moderate exercise is encouraged, but it's essential to consult with healthcare providers to ensure safety. Adequate hydration and sufficient rest are also essential components of a healthy pregnancy.

Prenatal care is a cornerstone of a healthy pregnancy. Regular check-ups with healthcare providers help monitor the baby's growth, detect potential issues early, and provide guidance on a healthy lifestyle.

Prenatal vitamins, recommended by healthcare professionals, aid in ensuring the mother and baby receive essential nutrients.

Emotional well-being is equally important during pregnancy. Hormonal changes, coupled with the anticipation of parenthood, can lead to mood swings and increased stress. Open communication with partners, family, and friends, as well as seeking support when needed, can contribute to a more positive pregnancy experience.

Childbirth education classes prepare expectant parents for labor, delivery, and postpartum care. These classes cover topics such as breathing techniques, pain management options, and newborn care basics. Understanding the birthing process empowers parents and reduces anxiety. Preparing for the baby's arrival involves creating a welcoming and safe environment. Setting up a nursery, attending prenatal classes, and acquiring essential baby gear are typical steps. Developing a birth plan detailing preferences for labor and delivery can also be beneficial.

However, pregnancy is a transformative and awe-inspiring journey that requires careful attention to both physical and emotional well-being. Educating oneself about the different stages, maintaining a healthy lifestyle, seeking prenatal care, and preparing for childbirth are essential components of a positive pregnancy experience. With proper care and support, expectant parents can navigate this incredible journey with confidence and joy, laying the foundation for a healthy start to their child's life.

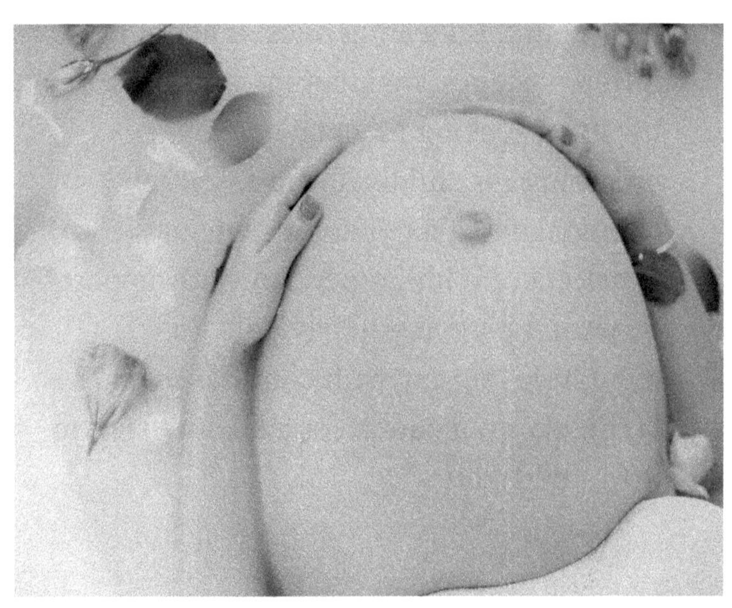

CHAPTER FOUR

ROLES OF DAD TO BE

The role of the father-to-be is a crucial and transformative one that extends beyond mere biological contribution. As a partner in the journey of parenthood, the father-to-be plays a significant role in the emotional, physical, and psychological well-being of both the expectant mother and the unborn child.

This role encompasses various dimensions, including providing support, fostering a healthy environment, and actively participating in the preparations for parenthood.

One of the primary responsibilities of the father-to-be is to offer emotional support to the expectant mother. Pregnancy is a time of profound physical and hormonal changes, and emotional support becomes paramount. The father-to-be can actively engage in open communication, expressing empathy, and being attuned to the emotional needs of the mother.

This support helps create a positive and secure environment for the mother, which is beneficial for her mental health and, consequently, the well-being of the developing fetus.

Moreover, the father-to-be plays a vital role in creating a healthy and supportive physical environment for the expectant mother. This involves participating in lifestyle changes that promote a positive pregnancy experience, such as maintaining a balanced diet, encouraging regular exercise, and creating a stress-free atmosphere.

By actively engaging in these aspects, the father-to-be contributes to the overall health and well-being of the expectant mother and the unborn child.

In addition to emotional and physical support, the father-to-be is instrumental in actively participating in the preparations for parenthood. This includes attending prenatal classes, reading parenting books, and educating oneself about the stages of pregnancy and childbirth.

By doing so, the father-to-be not only equips himself with the necessary knowledge but also demonstrates a commitment to shared responsibility in parenting.

As the due date approaches, the role of the father-to-be extends to being an advocate for the mother's needs during labor and childbirth. Providing a calming presence, offering encouragement, and communicating effectively with healthcare professionals are crucial aspects of this role.

The father-to-be's active involvement in the birthing process establishes a sense of partnership and shared responsibility, fostering a strong foundation for the parenting journey.

Beyond the immediate pre-birth period, the father-to-be continues to play a pivotal role in postpartum support. This involves actively participating in caregiving responsibilities, understanding the emotional and physical challenges of postpartum recovery, and ensuring a supportive and nurturing environment for both the mother and the newborn.

In essence, the role of the father-to-be is dynamic and multifaceted. It encompasses emotional support, active participation in physical well-being, and a commitment to shared responsibility in the journey of parenthood.

By embracing this role wholeheartedly, the father-to-be contributes significantly to the overall health and happiness of the family unit, setting the stage for a positive and fulfilling parenting experience.

CHAPTER FIVE

CHALLENGES OF PREGNANCY

Pregnancy is a remarkable and transformative period in a woman's life, marked by the development and nurturing of a new life within her. While it is a time of joy and anticipation, it also brings with it a multitude of challenges that can vary from woman to woman and pregnancy to pregnancy.

These challenges can be physical, emotional, and even social, making it essential for expectant mothers to receive proper support and care throughout this journey.

- Morning Sickness: Many women experience morning sickness during the first trimester, characterized by nausea and vomiting. While it usually subsides after the first trimester, it can be a challenging aspect of early pregnancy.

- Fatigue: Hormonal changes and the increased demands on the body during pregnancy often lead to fatigue. This can be particularly challenging for working women who may find it difficult to maintain their usual level of productivity.

- Body Changes: As the body adapts to accommodate the growing fetus, women may experience discomfort due to weight gain, changes in posture, and hormonal fluctuations. This can result in back pain, swollen ankles, and other physical discomforts.

- Mood Swings: Hormonal fluctuations can also impact a woman's emotional state, leading to mood swings. Women may find themselves

experiencing a range of emotions,
from joy and excitement to anxiety
and irritability.

- Body Image Concerns: The changes
in a woman's body during pregnancy
can sometimes lead to concerns about
body image. Society's expectations
and perceptions of beauty may
contribute to feelings of insecurity.

- Anxiety and Stress: The anticipation
of becoming a parent, coupled with
concerns about the health of the baby,
can contribute to increased anxiety
and stress levels. It's crucial for
pregnant women to have a strong
support system to help manage these
emotional challenges.

- Complications: Certain medical
conditions may arise during
pregnancy, such as gestational
diabetes, preeclampsia, or placenta
previa. These conditions require

careful monitoring and may necessitate changes in lifestyle or medical interventions.

- High-Risk Pregnancies: Some women are classified as having high-risk pregnancies due to pre-existing health conditions or complications that develop during pregnancy. This can lead to increased medical interventions and a need for specialized care.

- Workplace Issues: Balancing work responsibilities with the physical and emotional demands of pregnancy can be challenging. Some women may face discrimination or lack of understanding from employers and colleagues.

- Social Stigma: Cultural and societal expectations regarding pregnancy and motherhood can contribute to feelings of inadequacy or guilt, especially if the pregnancy was unplanned or if the woman faces challenges such as single parenthood.

- Cost of Prenatal Care: Medical expenses related to prenatal care, delivery, and postnatal care can be significant. Access to quality healthcare is essential, and financial constraints can add stress to an already challenging situation.

- Changes in Dynamics: The arrival of a baby often brings about changes in the dynamics of a relationship. It's important for couples to communicate openly and support each other during this transition.

- Sexual Intimacy: Physical changes and concerns about the well-being of the baby can impact sexual intimacy. Couples may need to navigate these changes together and find new ways to connect emotionally.

Pregnancy is a complex and multifaceted journey that involves physical, emotional, social, medical, financial, and relationship challenges. Each woman's experience is unique, and the level of difficulty can vary widely.

Adequate support from healthcare professionals, family, and friends, as well as open communication with a partner, can significantly contribute to a woman's well-being during this transformative time. Addressing these challenges collectively ensures a healthier and more positive pregnancy experience for both the mother and the baby.

CHAPTER SIX

IMPORTANCE OF PRENATAL VISITS

Prenatal visits are an essential aspect of prenatal care, providing a comprehensive framework for monitoring and promoting the health and well-being of both the pregnant woman and the developing fetus.

These visits involve a series of medical check-ups, screenings, and educational components that aim to ensure a healthy pregnancy and a positive outcome for both mother and baby.

Here's a comprehensive overview of prenatal visits:

**1. Initiation of Prenatal Care:
Early Engagement: Prenatal care ideally begins early in pregnancy, often during the

first trimester, as early care is associated with better outcomes.

Healthcare Provider: A healthcare provider, typically an obstetrician, midwife, or family physician, guides the expectant mother through the pregnancy journey.

**2. Frequency of Prenatal Visits:
Regular Appointments: Prenatal care involves a series of scheduled visits, typically spaced at regular intervals throughout the pregnancy.

Frequency Changes: The frequency of visits may vary based on individual health, gestational age, and any identified risk factors.

**3. Components of Prenatal Visits:
Medical Check-ups: Healthcare providers monitor vital signs, weight gain, blood pressure, and assess the overall health of the pregnant woman.

Fetal Monitoring: Fetal growth and development are tracked through techniques like ultrasound scans and Doppler monitoring of the baby's heartbeat.

Blood and Urine Tests: Routine blood tests check for conditions such as anemia, gestational diabetes, and infections. Urine tests may screen for conditions like preeclampsia.

**4. Screening for Complications:
Genetic Testing: Some prenatal visits include genetic screening to assess the risk of genetic disorders and birth defects.
Risk Assessment: Healthcare providers continually assess and manage any potential complications, adjusting the care plan accordingly.

**5. Educational Component:
Nutritional Guidance: Prenatal visits often include discussions on nutrition, vitamin supplementation, and healthy lifestyle choices.

Childbirth Education: Expectant parents receive information about the birthing process, pain management options, and postpartum care.

**6. Emotional Support:
Counseling: Prenatal visits may include discussions about emotional well-being, addressing any concerns or anxieties the expectant mother may have.

Partner Involvement: Partners are often encouraged to attend prenatal visits to enhance support and involvement in the pregnancy.

**7. Preparation for Labor and Delivery:
Birth Plans: Expectant parents can discuss and formulate birth plans, outlining preferences for labor and delivery.

Hospital Tours: Some prenatal programs include tours of birthing facilities to familiarize parents with the environment.

**8. Postpartum Planning:
Postpartum Care: Discussions about postpartum care and contraception options are often initiated during prenatal visits. Breastfeeding Support: Information and resources about breastfeeding are provided to prepare mothers for successful breastfeeding.

**9. Continuity of Care:
Communication: Prenatal visits facilitate open communication between the expectant parents and healthcare providers, fostering a supportive and collaborative relationship.

Monitoring Progress: The ongoing nature of prenatal care allows healthcare providers to monitor changes, address emerging issues, and adapt the care plan as needed.

**10. Emergency Preparedness:
Recognition of Warning Signs: Expectant mothers are educated about the signs and symptoms of complications, empowering

them to seek prompt medical attention if needed.

Prenatal visits play a crucial role in ensuring a healthy pregnancy by providing comprehensive medical care, emotional support, and education.

 Regular monitoring and early intervention contribute to the overall well-being of both the expectant mother and the developing fetus, laying the foundation for a positive childbirth experience and a healthy start for the newborn.

CHAPTER SEVEN

SEX DURING PREGNANCY

Sex during pregnancy is a topic that many expectant couples are curious about, and it's perfectly normal to have questions or concerns. Generally, it's important to note that a healthy pregnancy often allows for a continuation of sexual activity, provided there are no complications and both partners feel comfortable. However, it's crucial to consult with a healthcare professional for personalized advice based on the specific circumstances of the pregnancy.

Here are some key points to consider:

Communication is Key: Open and honest communication between partners is essential. Both individuals may have concerns or fears, and addressing them together can help alleviate any anxiety. It's important to share feelings, ask questions, and support each other emotionally.

Consultation with Healthcare Provider: Before engaging in sexual activity during pregnancy, it's advisable to consult with a healthcare provider. The healthcare professional can provide guidance based on the specific health of the pregnant person, the stage of the pregnancy, and any potential risk factors.

Normal Changes in Pregnancy: Pregnancy brings about various physical and hormonal changes in the body. These changes can affect sexual desire, comfort, and arousal. It's normal for libido to fluctuate, and physical changes such as breast tenderness, increased blood flow to the pelvic area, and changes in vaginal discharge are common.

Positioning and Comfort: As the pregnancy progresses, finding comfortable positions may become more challenging. Experimenting with different positions and finding what works best for both partners can enhance comfort. Many couples find side-by-side positions or those that allow the pregnant person to control the depth and pace to be comfortable.

Safety Concerns: In uncomplicated pregnancies, sexual activity is generally considered safe. However, if there are specific concerns, such as a history of miscarriage, preterm labor, or other complications, the healthcare provider may advise against certain activities. Conditions such as placenta previa or a weak cervix may necessitate additional precautions.

Benefits of Sex During Pregnancy

Engaging in sexual activity can have positive effects on the relationship. It helps maintain intimacy and emotional connection between partners during a time when the focus often shifts to the impending arrival of the baby. Additionally, sexual activity can promote relaxation and stress reduction.

Abstaining from Sex: In some cases, healthcare providers may recommend abstaining from sexual activity during certain stages of pregnancy. This might be due to specific complications or conditions. It's important to follow medical advice to ensure the health and well-being of both the pregnant person and the baby.

Please note that every pregnancy is unique, and what works for one couple may not be suitable for another. Consulting with a healthcare professional is crucial to receive personalized advice based on the specific circumstances of the pregnancy.

Ultimately, maintaining open communication, understanding each other's needs, and prioritizing comfort and safety are key factors in navigating sexual activity during pregnancy.

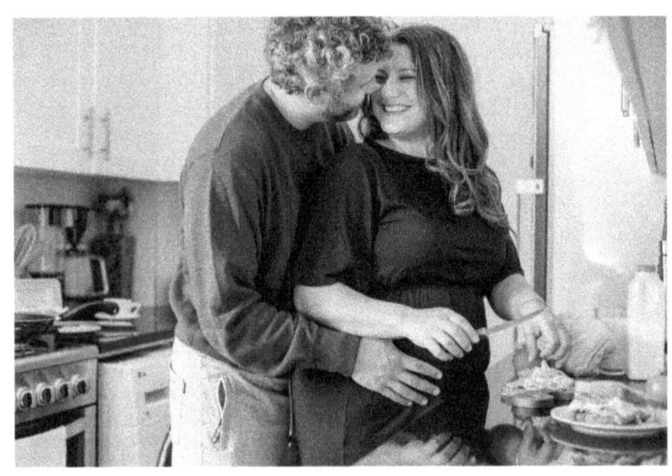

CHAPTER EIGHT

MORNING SICKNESS, PREGNANCY BRAIN AND CRAVING

Morning sickness is a common symptom experienced by many pregnant women, typically occurring during the first trimester of pregnancy. Contrary to the name, it can happen to a pregnant woman at any time of the day. Nausea and vomiting are the primary symptoms, and they can range from mild to severe.

The exact cause of morning sickness is not fully understood, but hormonal changes, especially the increase in human chorionic gonadotropin (hCG) during early pregnancy, are believed to play a role.

Managing morning sickness often involves lifestyle changes. Eating small, frequent meals and snacks, staying hydrated, and avoiding triggers like strong odors or certain foods can help alleviate symptoms. In some cases, healthcare providers may recommend vitamin B6 supplements or prescribe anti-nausea medications.

"Pregnancy brain" refers to cognitive changes that some pregnant women experience, such as forgetfulness, difficulty concentrating, and a feeling of mental fogginess. While the phenomenon is widely reported, scientific understanding is still evolving. Hormonal fluctuations, sleep disturbances, and the emotional and physical demands of pregnancy are thought to contribute.

It's important to note that these cognitive changes are typically temporary and resolve postpartum. Coping strategies include staying organized with lists and reminders, getting enough rest, and seeking support from friends and family.

Food cravings during pregnancy are a well-known phenomenon, and they can vary widely from person to person. These cravings often involve specific types of foods or unusual combinations. While the exact cause of pregnancy cravings is not fully understood, hormonal changes and nutritional needs are believed to be contributing factors.

Common cravings include sweet or salty foods, pickles, ice cream, and various fruits. It's generally considered safe to indulge in cravings in moderation, as long as they align with a balanced and nutritious diet.

However, if cravings involve non-food items (a condition known as pica), it's crucial to consult a healthcare professional, as this may indicate a nutritional deficiency.

Pregnancy is a unique and individual experience, and each woman may encounter these symptoms to varying degrees.

Seeking regular prenatal care, maintaining a healthy lifestyle, and communicating openly with healthcare providers can help address and manage these aspects of pregnancy.

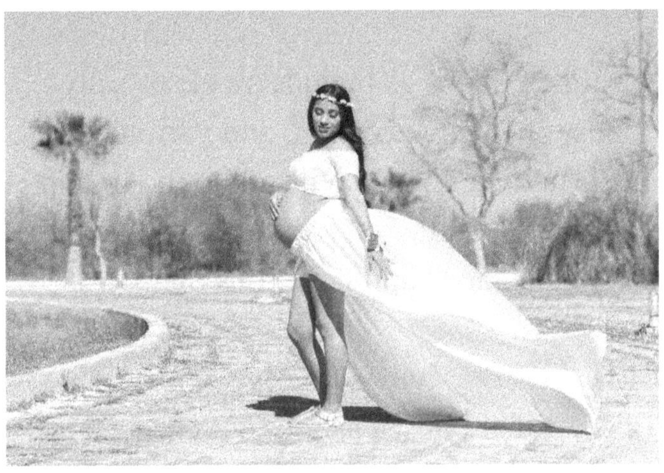

CHAPTER NINE

EXPECTATIONS FOR A MODERN DAD

Modern dads are breaking away from traditional stereotypes and embracing a more active and involved role in parenting. The expectations for a modern dad have evolved to reflect the changing dynamics of families, gender roles, and societal norms.

 Here are some key expectations for a modern dad:

- Active Parenting: Modern dads are expected to be actively involved in all aspects of parenting, from diaper changing to school activities. They share responsibilities with the mother and actively participate in childcare, ensuring a more balanced and equitable division of labor.

- Emotional Support: A modern dad is not just a provider but also an emotional anchor for the family. He is expected to be emotionally supportive, understanding, and communicative. Building strong emotional connections with his children is considered essential for their overall well-being.

- Work-Life Balance: Striking a healthy work-life balance is crucial for modern dads. They are expected to prioritize family time, be present for important events, and find ways to manage their professional commitments without sacrificing their role as a parent.

- Inclusivity and Equality: Modern dads are expected to promote gender equality within the family. This includes challenging traditional gender roles, treating all family members with respect, and actively participating in discussions and decisions related to parenting and household responsibilities.

- Role Modeling: Being a positive role model is a significant expectation for modern dads. They are expected to demonstrate qualities such as empathy, responsibility, and resilience, teaching their children by example about the values that are important in life.

- Flexibility: Modern dads need to be flexible and adaptable. Parenting often comes with unexpected challenges, and the ability to adjust plans, routines, and expectations is essential for navigating the complexities of family life.

- Learning and Growing: A modern dad is expected to be open to learning and growing as a parent. Keeping up with the latest parenting trends, understanding child development, and continuously improving parenting skills are important aspects of being a modern and informed father.

- Supporting Career Ambitions: Modern dads support not only their children's dreams but also those of their partners. They encourage their children to pursue their passions and support their partners in achieving their career goals.

- Technology Literacy: With the increasing role of technology in education and daily life, modern dads are expected to be tech-savvy. This includes helping with homework that involves technology, monitoring online activities, and guiding their children in the responsible use of digital resources.

- Self-Care: Taking care of one's physical and mental well-being is a priority for modern dads. Recognizing the importance of self-care sets an example for their children and contributes to a healthier family dynamic.

In essence, the expectations for a modern dad revolve around being actively engaged, emotionally present, and adaptable in the ever-changing landscape of parenting and family life. Embracing these expectations contributes to the development of healthier, more balanced, and connected families.

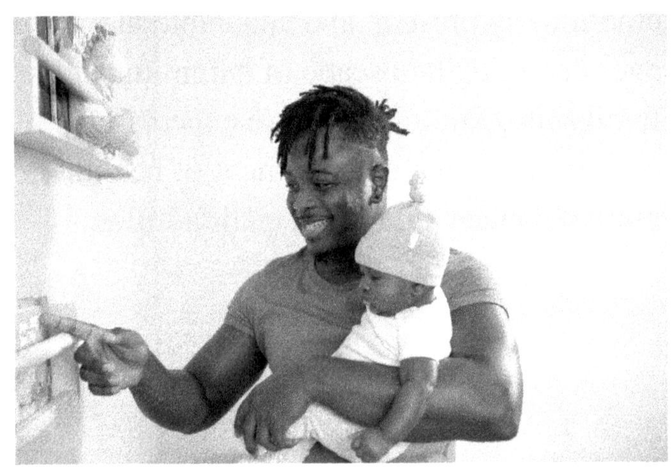

CHAPTER TEN

MAINTAINING HEALTH AND WELLNESS

Maintaining health and wellness during pregnancy is crucial for the well-being of both the mother and the developing baby. Here are some key guidelines to help ensure a healthy and positive pregnancy experience.

Regular Prenatal Check-ups:Always schedule and attend regular prenatal check-ups with your healthcare professional. These visits help monitor the progress of your pregnancy and address any potential issues early on.

Balanced Diet:Always consume a well-balanced diet that includes many fruits, vegetables, whole grains, lean proteins, and dairy products as proper nutrition is essential for the growth and development of the baby.

Adequate Hydration:Always drink plenty of water throughout the day to stay hydrated as water is crucial for maintaining amniotic fluid levels and supporting the increased blood volume during pregnancy.

Supplements:Try to take prenatal vitamins and supplements as recommended by your healthcare provider. These may include folic acid, iron, calcium, and other nutrients essential for fetal development.

Regular Exercise:Engage in moderate and safe exercises suitable for pregnant women. Activities like walking, swimming, and prenatal yoga can help maintain physical fitness, reduce discomfort, and promote a healthy pregnancy.

Adequate Rest:Ensure you get enough sleep and rest. Fatigue is common during pregnancy, and getting sufficient rest is vital for the body to recover and for the overall well-being of both the mother and the baby.

Stress Management:Practice stress-reducing techniques such as meditation, deep breathing, and prenatal yoga. Chronic stress can negatively impact both maternal and fetal health.

Avoid Harmful Substances:Steer clear of alcohol, tobacco, and recreational drugs. Try to limit caffeine intake and avoid exposure to harmful chemicals and environmental toxins stuffs.

Educate Yourself:Attend prenatal classes to gain knowledge about childbirth, breastfeeding, and newborn care. Being informed can help alleviate anxiety and empower you to make informed decisions.

Dental Care:Always maintain good and proper oral hygiene by regularly brushing and flossing your teeth. Hormonal changes during pregnancy can increase the risk of gum disease, so dental care is crucial.

Weight Management:Aim for healthy weight gain during pregnancy. Your healthcare provider can guide you on the appropriate weight gain based on your pre-pregnancy BMI.

Social Support:Always surround yourself with a supportive network of family, colleagues and friends. Emotional well-being is just as important as physical health during pregnancy.

Steer clear of bad habits:Reduce your exposure to secondhand smoke and give up smoking. Cut back on alcohol intake or stay away from it completely.

Sanitation and Hygiene:Maintain proper hygiene, which includes frequent hand washing, to stop the spread of illnesses. Keeping your home clean will help you be less exposed to irritants and pollutants.

Social Network: Keep up a solid support system of friends and family by cultivating strong social relationships.
Take part in events that encourage community building and social engagement.

Set Achievable Health Goals: Make sure your health objectives are time-bound, quantifiable, and explicit.
To keep yourself motivated, acknowledge and appreciate your little victories along the road.

Positivity: Develop an optimistic outlook and practice thankfulness.
Pay attention to the areas of your life that make you happy and fulfilled.
Recall that maintaining your health requires taking care of your physical, mental, and emotional needs. Long-term improvements to your general health can be achieved with consistent work and dedication to a healthy lifestyle.

Remember to consult with your healthcare provider before making any significant lifestyle changes, as individual health needs can vary. By prioritizing these aspects of health and wellness, you can contribute to a positive and healthy pregnancy journey.

CHAPTER ELEVEN

BODY CHANGES

Pregnancy is a transformative journey for a woman, marked by numerous physical and physiological changes as her body adapts to support the growth and development of a new life.

These changes are a result of complex hormonal fluctuations and the demands of nurturing a developing fetus. Here are some of the key body changes that occur during pregnancy.

Weight Gain: Weight gain is a natural and essential aspect of pregnancy. The average weight gain recommended by healthcare providers varies depending on pre-pregnancy weight, but it generally falls within a specific range. This weight gain includes the baby, placenta, amniotic fluid, increased blood volume, and enlarged uterus.

Enlarged Breasts: Hormonal changes cause the breasts to become larger, tender, and more sensitive. This prepares the body for breastfeeding by increasing blood flow and expanding mammary glands.

Skin Changes: Pregnancy hormones, particularly estrogen, can affect the skin. Some women experience a pregnancy glow due to increased blood flow, while others may develop dark patches (melasma) or a dark line running from the belly button to the pubic area (linea nigra). Stretch marks may also appear as the skin stretches to accommodate the growing belly.

Changes in Hair and Nails: Hormonal fluctuations can impact hair growth. Some women may experience thicker, shinier hair during pregnancy, while others may notice changes in texture. Sometimes nails may grow faster and become stronger.
Swelling and Fluid Retention: Increased blood volume and hormonal changes can

lead to fluid retention, causing swelling in the hands, feet, and ankles. This is a common discomfort during pregnancy.

Changes in the Cardiovascular System: The heart has to work harder to pump the increased volume of blood throughout the body. This can lead to an elevated heart rate and, in some cases, changes in blood pressure.

Digestive System Changes: Hormonal influences can affect the digestive system, leading to symptoms such as heartburn, constipation, and nausea, especially during the first trimester.

Enlarged Uterus: As the fetus grows, the uterus expands to accommodate the developing baby. This can cause a visible change in the shape and size of the abdomen.

Joint and Ligament Relaxation: Hormones like relaxin cause joints and ligaments to become more flexible. While this is essential for accommodating the growing baby and preparing for childbirth, it can also result in increased susceptibility to joint-related discomfort.

Changes in the Reproductive Organs: The cervix and vagina undergo changes during pregnancy, and increased blood flow to the pelvic region is common. These changes prepare the body for labor and delivery.

It's important to note that each woman's experience of pregnancy is unique, and while these changes are common, the degree and timing of these changes can vary.

Regular prenatal care and communication with healthcare providers are crucial for monitoring and addressing any concerns during this transformative period.

CHAPTER TWELVE

FIRST TRIMESTER

The first trimester of pregnancy is a crucial time for both the mother and the developing fetus. Here are some important things to see and consider during this period.

Prenatal Care:Try to schedule your first prenatal appointment as soon as you confirm that you are pregnant.
Regular check-ups are important for monitoring the health of both the mother and the child.

Healthy Lifestyle:Maintain a well-balanced diet with a focus on prenatal vitamins containing folic acid.Avoid alcohol, smoking, and illicit drugs. Limit caffeine intake. Stay hydrated.

Rest and Sleep:Ensure you get enough rest and sleep to support your body and the developing baby.

Symptoms and Discomfort:Understand and manage common symptoms like morning sickness, fatigue, and mood swings. Consult with your healthcare provider about safe remedies for alleviating discomfort.

Exercise:Engage in moderate and safe exercises, as advised by your healthcare provider. Yoga and walking are often recommended during the first trimester.

Work Environment:If your job involves exposure to harmful substances or physical strain, discuss potential adjustments with your employer.

Avoid Certain Foods:Be aware of foods that may pose a risk during pregnancy, such as raw fish, unpasteurized dairy, and certain types of deli meats.

Genetic Testing and Screenings:Discuss with your healthcare provider about genetic testing and screenings that may be recommended based on your medical history and family background.

Educate Yourself:Take prenatal classes to learn about pregnancy, childbirth, and postpartum care.Read reliable pregnancy books and resources to stay informed.

Emotional Well-being:Be aware of your emotional health and seek support if needed. Try to join support groups or talk to friends, colleagues, and family about your feelings and concerns.

Financial Planning:Start planning for the financial aspects of pregnancy and childbirth, including insurance coverage and potential medical expenses.

Plan for Maternity Leave:If you are working, discuss maternity leave options with your employer and plan accordingly.

Fetal Development:Understand the stages of fetal development and follow the growth of your baby through ultrasound appointments.

Infections and Vaccinations:Be cautious about exposure to infections and discuss with your healthcare provider about vaccinations that are safe during pregnancy.

Plan for Baby's Arrival:Begin planning for the baby's arrival by setting up a nursery, choosing a healthcare provider for the baby, and making necessary preparations. Always consult with your healthcare provider for personalized advice and guidance based on your individual health and pregnancy.

Every pregnancy is unique, and your healthcare team can provide the best recommendations for your specific situation.

CHAPTER THIRTEEN

BABY AT FIRST TRIMESTER

The first trimester of pregnancy is a crucial period of development for the growing embryo. Here are some major milestones and changes that occur to both mother and child during the first trimester.

Fertilization and Implantation (Week 1-2): The first trimester begins with fertilization of the egg by sperm, forming a zygote.

The zygote then undergoes several cell divisions as it travels down the fallopian tube. By the end of the first week, it develops into a blastocyst. Around the end of the second week, the blastocyst attaches to the uterine lining in a process called implantation.

Formation of Germ Layers (Week 3-4): During the third and fourth weeks, the blastocyst differentiates into three germ layers – ectoderm, mesoderm, and endoderm.

These three layers do give rise to various organs and tissues.
Development of Major Organs and Structures (Week 5-8): By the fifth week, the neural tube begins to form, which eventually becomes the brain and spinal cord. Also, at this point the heart starts beating and limb buds will appear. Major organs such as the heart, lungs, liver, and kidneys begin to take shape. Facial features also start to form.

Placenta and Umbilical Cord (Week 6-10): The placenta, which provides nutrients and oxygen to the developing fetus, begins to develop around the sixth week. The umbilical cord, connecting the baby to the placenta, forms during this time.

Fetal Movement (Week 8-12): While the mother may not feel it, the fetus starts making spontaneous movements around the eighth week. However, these movements are generally too small to be detected by the mother.

Sexual Differentiation (Week 9-12): The fetus's sexual organs continue to develop, and by the end of the first trimester, it is possible to identify the baby's sex through ultrasound.

End of the First Trimester (Week 12): By the end of the 12th week, the first trimester concludes, and the developing baby is referred to as a fetus. At this point, most of the major organ systems have formed, and the risk of miscarriage significantly decreases.

It's important to note that the first trimester is a critical time, and exposure to harmful substances (such as certain medications, alcohol, and tobacco) during this period can have significant effects on fetal development.

Regular prenatal care is essential to monitor the health and progress of both the mother and the developing baby.

CHAPTER FOURTEEN

MOTHER AT FIRST TRIMESTER

The first trimester of pregnancy is a crucial and dynamic period during which significant changes occur in both the mother's body and the developing fetus. Here are some key aspects of what happens to the mother during the first trimester.

Hormonal Changes:The body experiences a surge in hormones, particularly human chorionic gonadotropin (hCG), progesterone, and estrogen.

These hormonal changes help maintain the uterine lining, support the placenta, and prevent the shedding of the uterine lining, which would result in a miscarriage.

Physical Changes:Many women experience symptoms such as morning sickness (nausea and vomiting), fatigue, breast tenderness, and frequent urination.

At this stage, the uterus begins to expand to accommodate the growing fetus.

Some women may notice changes in their skin, such as darkening of the areolas and the appearance of a linea nigra (a dark line that runs down the abdomen).

Development of the Placenta:The placenta starts to form and take over the production of hormones to support the pregnancy.
It serves as a vital link between the mother and the developing fetus, providing nutrients and oxygen while removing waste products.

Fetal Development:During the first trimester, the major organs and systems of the developing fetus begin to form. By the end of the first trimester, the fetus has developed all major organs, and its basic structure is in place.The heartbeat becomes detectable, and the fetus goes through rapid growth and development.

Emotional Changes:Many women experience a range of emotions during the first trimester, which can include excitement, anxiety, and mood swings. Hormonal fluctuations and the realization of the impending changes in life contribute to these emotional changes.

Medical Monitoring:Women typically have regular prenatal check-ups to monitor the progress of the pregnancy, ensure the well-being of both the mother and the fetus, and address any concerns or complications that may arise.

It's important to note that every pregnancy is unique, and not all women will experience the same symptoms or changes during the first trimester.

Additionally, while some discomforts are common, severe symptoms or complications should be discussed with a healthcare provider for appropriate guidance and care.

Regular prenatal care is crucial to ensuring a healthy pregnancy and addressing any issues that may arise.

CHAPTER FIFTEEN

A MUST-KNOW-FOR NEW MOMS

The first trimester of pregnancy is a crucial and exciting time, as it marks the beginning of the development of the baby and significant changes in the mother's body. Here are some key points that a new mom should know about the first trimester.

Confirming Pregnancy:Always confirm your pregnancy with a home pregnancy tcst or you visit your healthcare provider.

Prenatal Care:Try to schedule your first prenatal appointment with a healthcare provider. Regular prenatal care is essential for monitoring the health of both you and your baby.

Nutrition:Focus on a balanced diet rich in nutrients, including folic acid, iron, calcium, and other essential vitamins and minerals. Stay hydrated and try to avoid excessive caffeine intake.

Folic Acid:Take a prenatal vitamin with folic acid to help prevent neural tube defects in the developing baby.

Morning Sickness:Many women experience morning sickness, which may occur at any time of the day depending on the individual. Eat small, frequent meals, and stay hydrated to help manage nausea.

Fatigue:It's normal to feel more tired during the first trimester. Always listen to your body system and get plenty of rest.

Avoid Harmful Substances:During pregnancy, avoid alcohol, tobacco, and illicit drugs, as they can harm the developing baby.

Medications:Inform your healthcare provider about any medications you are taking, as some may not be safe during pregnancy.

Exercise:Stay active with moderate exercise, but consult your healthcare provider before starting a new exercise routine.

Emotional Well-being:Pregnancy hormones can affect your emotions. It's normal to experience mood swings. Seek support from your partner, friends, or a healthcare professional if needed.

Sleep:Ensure you get enough sleep, and consider sleeping on your side to improve blood flow to the baby.

Body Changes:You may experience breast tenderness, changes in skin pigmentation, and increased urination.

Ultrasound and Screening Tests:Your healthcare provider may recommend ultrasound and other screening tests to assess the health of the baby.

Educate Yourself:Learn about the changes happening in your body and the development of your baby. Attend prenatal classes if available.

Work:Inform your employer about your pregnancy, and discuss any necessary workplace adjustments with your healthcare provider.

It's essential to communicate openly with your healthcare provider about any concerns or questions you may have. They can provide personalized advice based on your health and the needs of your pregnancy.

CHAPTER SIXTEEN

SECOND TRIMESTER AND ITS CHALLENGES

The second trimester of pregnancy, spanning from weeks 13 to 28, is often referred to as the "honeymoon phase" for many expectant mothers.

During this period, the initial challenges of the first trimester, such as morning sickness and fatigue, tend to subside, and women often experience a surge in energy and an improved sense of well-being.

However, the second trimester does come with its own set of challenges:

Growing Belly and Body Changes: As the baby continues to grow, the mother's abdomen expands, and she may start to feel the physical effects of carrying extra weight. This can lead to backaches, increased pressure on the pelvis, and changes in posture, causing discomfort and fatigue.

Stretch Marks and Skin Changes: The rapid growth of the belly during the second trimester can result in stretch marks as the skin stretches to accommodate the growing baby. Hormonal changes may also lead to pigmentation changes, such as the development of the linea nigra (a dark line on the abdomen) and melasma (darkening of facial skin).

Varied Emotional Experiences: While the hormonal fluctuations and emotional ups and downs of the first trimester may stabilize, the second trimester can bring a mix of emotions. Some women may feel more emotionally balanced, while others may experience mood swings or anxiety about the impending responsibilities of motherhood.

Increased Appetite and Weight Gain: Many women find that their appetite increases during the second trimester. While it's important to nourish both the mother and the developing baby, excessive weight gain can pose health risks. Striking a balance between providing adequate nutrition and maintaining a healthy weight becomes crucial.

Fetal Movement and Sleep Disturbances: The baby's movements become more pronounced during the second trimester, which is a positive sign of healthy development. However, these movements can sometimes interfere with the mother's ability to sleep, causing disturbances during the night.

Gestational Diabetes Screening: Around 24 to 28 weeks, healthcare providers typically screen pregnant women for gestational diabetes. This condition can develop during pregnancy and may require dietary changes, monitoring blood sugar levels, or medication to manage.

Anatomy Scan and Potential Challenges: The second trimester often includes an anatomy scan, a detailed ultrasound examination to check the baby's growth and development. While most pregnancies progress smoothly, some may reveal potential challenges or abnormalities, requiring further evaluation and decisions.

Preparation for Labor and Delivery: As the due date approaches, expectant mothers may start thinking more about labor and delivery. This can be accompanied by a mix of excitement, anticipation, and anxiety. Attending childbirth classes and making birth plans become common activities during this phase.

It's essential for expectant mothers to stay in regular communication with their healthcare providers, address any concerns promptly, and prioritize self-care during the second trimester.

Individual experiences may vary, so seeking guidance and support from healthcare professionals, friends, and family can be invaluable during this transformative time.

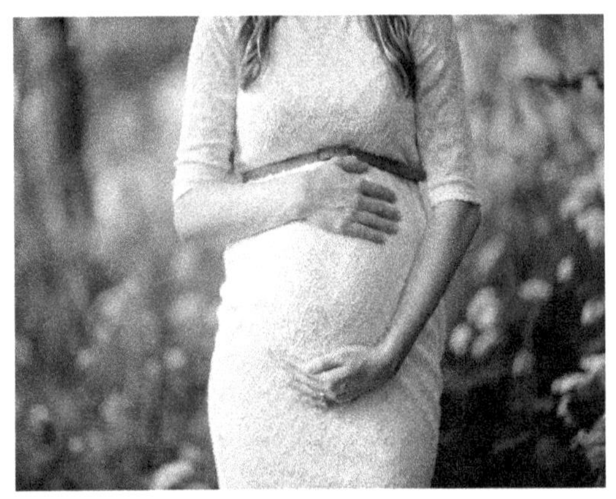

CHAPTER SEVENTEEN

DO THIS IN SECOND TRIMESTER

Congratulations to the new parents! The second trimester of pregnancy is often considered the "golden period" because many women experience relief from the initial symptoms of pregnancy.

Here are some things that new parents can consider during the second trimester:

Prenatal Care:Continue attending regular prenatal check-ups with the healthcare provider.Always discuss any concerns or questions with the healthcare professional.

Healthy Lifestyle:Maintain a balanced and nutritious diet, including foods rich in folic acid, iron, and calcium.Stay hydrated by drinking plenty of water.Continue taking prenatal vitamins as recommended by the healthcare provider.

Exercise:Engage in regular, moderate exercise with the approval of the healthcare provider. Prenatal yoga or swimming can be good options.
Exercise can help with overall well-being, reduce stress, and promote better sleep.

Baby Bump Bonding:Attend ultrasound appointments to see the baby's development and hear the heartbeat.
Consider scheduling a 3D or 4D ultrasound for a more detailed view of the baby.

Educate Yourselves:Always attend prenatal classes to learn about pregnancy, childbirth, breastfeeding, and newborn care.Read books or take online courses about pregnancy, childbirth, and parenting.

Prepare for Baby:Start planning the baby's nursery and collecting necessary baby items.Look into birthing options and create a birth plan.

Connect with Other Parents:Join local or online parenting groups to connect with other expectant parents.Share experiences and seek advice from others who have been through similar situations.

Emotional Well-being:Take time for self-care and relaxation.
Communicate openly with each other about expectations and concerns.
Consider attending prenatal counseling or support groups if needed.

Capture the Moment:Document the pregnancy journey through photos and journaling.

Consider a maternity photoshoot to capture the memories.

Plan Maternity Leave and Parental Leave: plan maternity and paternal leave with employers.
Explore your company's policies and ensure necessary paperwork is in order.

It's important for parents to listen to their bodies and communicate openly with healthcare providers. If any concerns or questions arise, don't hesitate to reach out to the healthcare team for guidance and support.

CHAPTER EIGHTEEN

DEALING WITH WEIGHT LOSS AND WEIGHT GAIN

Pregnancy is a unique time in a woman's life, and both weight loss and weight gain can be common experiences.

It's important to approach these changes in a healthy and balanced way, keeping the well-being of both the mother and the developing baby in mind. Always consult with your healthcare provider before making any significant changes to your diet or exercise routine during pregnancy.

Follow a Balanced Diet:Eat a variety of nutrient-rich foods, including fruits, vegetables, whole grains, lean proteins, and dairy products.Focus on proper portion sizes to avoid excessive calorie intake.Stay hydrated by drinking plenty of water.

Regular Prenatal Check-ups:Attend regular prenatal appointments to monitor your weight gain and receive guidance from your healthcare provider.They can help you set appropriate weight gain goals based on your pre-pregnancy weight and overall health.

Moderate Exercise:Engage in moderate exercise if your healthcare provider approves. Activities like walking, swimming, and prenatal yoga can be beneficial.Exercise can help control weight gain, improve mood, and promote overall well-being.

Listen to Your Body:Pay attention to hunger and fullness cues by avoiding eating emotionally but focus on nourishing your body with balanced and healthy foods.

Educate Yourself:Understand that weight gain is a natural part of a healthy pregnancy. Aim for steady, gradual weight gain rather than drastic changes.

Consult Your Healthcare Provider:If you're experiencing unintended weight loss during pregnancy, it's crucial to speak with your healthcare provider promptly.
They help in identifying the underlying causes and provide appropriate guidance.

Focus on Nutrient-Dense Foods:Choose foods that are rich in nutrients to ensure you and your baby are getting essential vitamins and minerals.
Consider consulting a nutritionist for personalized advice.

Small, Frequent Meals:Eating smaller, more frequent meals can help if you're experiencing nausea or have difficulty eating large portions.

Stay Hydrated:Drink plenty of water to stay hydrated, especially if you're experiencing vomiting or loss of appetite.

Rest and Self-Care:Ensure you're getting enough rest to support your body during this demanding time.

Manage stress through activities like relaxation exercises, meditation, or prenatal yoga.

Please note that every pregnancy is unique and individual circumstances also vary. Always consult your healthcare provider for personalized advice tailored to your specific needs and health conditions.

CHAPTER NINETEEN

UNTOLD SECRETS

The second trimester of pregnancy spans from weeks 13 to 27. During this period, significant developments occur in the baby's growth and development. Here are some key milestones and changes that take place during the second trimester.

Fetal Development

Organs and Systems: The baby's organs and systems continue to develop. By the end of the second trimester, most of the major organs are formed, and they start functioning.

Movement: The baby begins to move actively. While the mother may not feel strong movements early in the second trimester, by the later weeks, she is likely to feel distinct kicks and flutters.

Appearance

Facial Features: Facial features become more defined. Eyebrows and eyelashes develop, and the baby's face starts to look more human-like.

Vernix and Lanugo: A fine layer of hair called lanugo and a waxy substance called vernix caseosa form on the baby's skin. These substances protect the skin and provide insulation.

Sensory Development

Sensory Organs: The baby's sensory organs, such as the eyes and ears, continue to develop. By the end of the second trimester, the baby can hear sounds from the outside world.

Gender Identification: In most cases, the baby's gender can be identified during the second trimester through ultrasound.

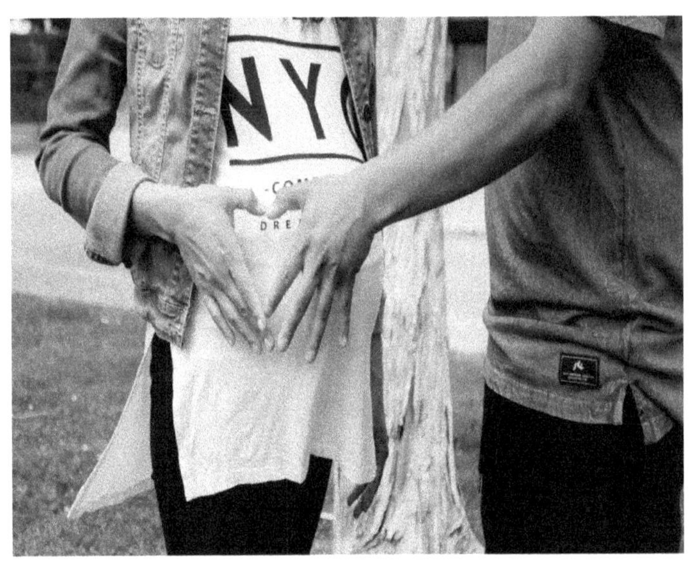

CHAPTER TWENTY

HORMONAL SHIFT

During the second trimester of pregnancy, which spans from weeks 13 to 28, various hormonal changes continue to play a crucial role in supporting the growth and development of the fetus. Some of the key hormonal shifts during this period include:

Human Chorionic Gonadotropin (hCG): While hCG is highest in the first trimester, it continues to be produced throughout pregnancy. It helps maintain the corpus luteum, which, in turn, produces progesterone during the early stages of pregnancy.

Progesterone: Produced by the corpus luteum and later by the placenta, progesterone helps maintain the uterine lining and supports the implantation of the embryo. It continues to rise during the second trimester, contributing to the development of the placenta and preventing contractions that could lead to preterm labor.

Estrogen: Estrogen levels increase significantly during the second trimester, primarily produced by the placenta. This hormone plays a vital role in the development of the fetus, the growth of the placenta, and the preparation of the breasts for breastfeeding.

Prolactin: Produced by the pituitary gland, prolactin levels gradually increase during pregnancy. While its primary role is to stimulate milk production in preparation for breastfeeding, high levels during pregnancy also contribute to changes in breast tissue.

Human Placental Lactogen (hPL): This hormone, produced by the placenta, helps regulate maternal metabolism to ensure a steady supply of nutrients to the developing fetus. It also plays the vital role of preparing the breasts for lactation.

Cortisol: Produced by the adrenal glands, cortisol levels increase during pregnancy. This hormone is essential for fetal organ development and helps regulate the immune system.

Insulin: Insulin sensitivity decreases during pregnancy, leading to an increase in insulin production. This helps ensure an adequate supply of glucose to support fetal growth.

Thyroid Hormones: Thyroid hormone levels may increase during pregnancy. These hormones are crucial for the development of the baby's brain and nervous system.

Overall, these hormonal shifts work together to create a supportive environment for the growing fetus and prepare the mother's body for childbirth and breastfeeding.

It's important to note that individual variations exist, and hormonal changes can affect women differently during pregnancy. If you have specific concerns about your pregnancy, it's always best to consult with your healthcare provider for personalized guidance and information.

CHAPTER TWENTY-ONE

NEW MOM AND DAD

The second trimester of pregnancy is often considered the "honeymoon phase" as many women experience a decrease in early pregnancy symptoms like nausea and fatigue. It's a great time for expectant parents to prepare for the arrival of their baby. Here are some things new moms and dads can do during the second trimester:

Attend Prenatal Classes:Consider taking prenatal classes to learn about childbirth, breastfeeding, and newborn care. These classes can help both parents feel more prepared and confident.

Schedule and Attend Medical Check-ups: Keep up with regular prenatal check-ups and ultrasounds. This is an important time for monitoring the baby's development and addressing any concerns.

Create a Birth Plan:Discuss and create a birth plan with your healthcare provider. This can include preferences for pain management, delivery positions, and other aspects of labor and delivery.

Investigate Childcare Options:If both parents plan to return to work after the baby is born, start researching and visiting potential childcare options. It's never too early to secure a spot if necessary.

Plan the Nursery:Begin planning and setting up the nursery. This can include choosing a color scheme, selecting furniture, and getting organized with baby essentials.

Attend Parenting Classes: Consider classes on parenting skills and infant CPR. These can provide valuable information and boost confidence in caring for a newborn.

Discuss Parental Leave:Have a conversation with your employer about parental leave options. Be sure to understand your rights and make any necessary arrangements for time off after the baby is born.

Exercise and Stay Active:As a pregnant woman always engage in moderate exercise with your healthcare professional's approval. Prenatal yoga, swimming, and walking are often recommended to maintain fitness and alleviate discomfort.

Connect with Other Expectant Parents: Join prenatal groups or classes to connect with other expectant parents. Sharing experiences and building a support network can be valuable.

Plan a Babymoon:Consider taking a babymoon, a relaxing getaway before the baby arrives. Make sure to choose a destination and activities that are safe during pregnancy.

Have open and honest discussions about parenting roles, responsibilities, and expectations. This is a good time to align on parenting philosophies and goals.

Research Pediatricians:Begin researching and selecting a pediatrician for your baby. Schedule a meeting with potential pediatricians to discuss their approach and ask any questions you may have.

It is essential to communicate openly with each other and with healthcare providers. Preparing for parenthood is a gradual process, and taking these steps during the second trimester can help ease the transition into becoming parents.

CHAPTER TWENTY-TWO

THIRD TRIMESTER OVERVIEW

The third trimester of pregnancy is the final phase, spanning from week 28 until the birth of the baby, typically around week 40. This trimester is marked by significant growth and development of the fetus, as well as changes in the mother's body in preparation for childbirth. These are some major aspects third trimester:

Fetal Development:The fetus undergoes rapid growth during the third trimester. Organs and systems that have developed in earlier trimesters continue to mature. The baby's lungs develop further, preparing for breathing outside the womb.

The baby gains significant weight, and there is a marked increase in fat deposition under the skin.

Maternal Changes:The mother's abdomen continues to expand as the baby grows, and the uterus extends upward toward the ribcage.Women may experience increased back pain, pelvic pressure, and discomfort due to the extra weight and pressure on the pelvic area.Changes in hormone levels may lead to symptoms such as heartburn, indigestion, and swelling in the extremities.

Braxton Hicks Contractions: Women may experience practice contractions known as Braxton Hicks contractions. These are basically sporadic irregular contractions that help prepare the uterus for labor.

Breast Changes:The breasts continue to undergo changes in preparation for breastfeeding. They may become larger, more tender, and produce colostrum, a precursor to breast milk.

Increased Urination:Pressure on the bladder from the growing uterus may lead to more frequent urination.

Nesting Instinct:Some women experience a "nesting" instinct, where they have a burst of energy and an urge to prepare for the baby's arrival by organizing and cleaning their living space.

Preparation for Labor:As the due date approaches, the baby usually moves into a head-down position in preparation for birth. At this point, the cervix on its own will begin to soften, thin out (efface), and open (dilate) in preparation for labor. However, this process is called "cervical ripening".

Medical Checkups:Regular prenatal checkups become more frequent in the third trimester. Healthcare providers monitor the baby's position, growth, and the overall health of both the mother and baby.

Tests such as Group B streptococcus (GBS) screening may be performed, and the provider discusses the birth plan with the expectant mother.

It's good for pregnant individuals to maintain a healthy lifestyle, get adequate rest, and communicate any concerns or unusual symptoms to their healthcare provider during the third trimester. As the due date approaches, it's also common for expectant parents to attend childbirth education classes to prepare for labor, delivery, and the early postpartum period.

CHAPTER TWENTY-THREE

GETTING PASS THIRD TRIMESTER

The term "third trimester" is typically associated with pregnancy, referring to the final three months of gestation. If you're asking about getting through the third trimester of pregnancy, here are some general tips:

Regular Prenatal Care: Ensure you attend all your prenatal check-ups. Regular medical check-ups are crucial for monitoring the health of both you and your baby.

Healthy Diet: Maintain a balanced and nutritious diet. Consume foods rich in vitamins, minerals, and nutrients necessary for the development of your baby.

Hydration: Stay well-hydrated by drinking plenty of water. Proper hydration is essential for your health and the well-being of your baby.

Rest and Sleep: Get adequate rest and sleep. As you progress through the third trimester, you may find it more challenging to get comfortable at night, so try using pillows for support.

Exercise: Engage in gentle and approved exercises for pregnant women. Activities like walking and swimming can help with circulation and reduce discomfort.

Pelvic Exercises: Consider doing pelvic floor exercises to prepare for labor and reduce the risk of complications.

Educate Yourself: Attend childbirth education classes to learn about the birthing process and postpartum care.

Prepare for Labor: Pack your hospital bag, plan your transportation to the hospital or birthing center, and discuss your birthing preferences with your healthcare provider.

Communicate with Your Healthcare Provider: Keep open communication with your healthcare provider about any concerns, changes, or symptoms you may be experiencing.

Emotional Well-being: Pay attention to your emotional well-being. Pregnancy can bring about various emotions, so ensure you have a support system in place.
If your question is not related to pregnancy, please provide more context so that I can better assist you.

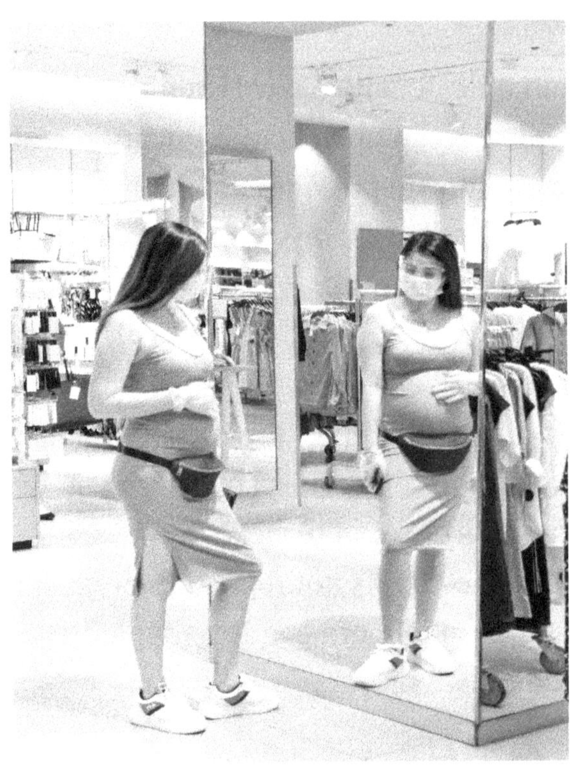

CHAPTER TWENTY-FOUR

BABY AT THIRD TRIMESTER

During the third trimester of pregnancy, which spans from weeks 28 to 40, significant development and preparation occur as the baby gets ready for birth. Here are some key aspects of fetal development and changes that happen during the third trimester:

Fetal Growth: The baby experiences rapid growth, gaining more weight and developing fat deposits that help regulate body temperature after birth.

Organ Development: Most of the baby's organs are fully formed by the end of the second trimester, but during the third trimester, they continue to mature and develop further.

Lung Development: The lungs go through important developments to become capable of functioning outside the womb. Surfactant, a substance that helps the air sacs in the lungs stay open, is produced in increasing amounts.

Brain Development: The brain undergoes further development, including the formation of more intricate neural connections and the accumulation of essential nutrients for brain growth.

Movement and Positioning: The baby becomes more active and usually assumes a head-down position in preparation for birth.

However, some babies may be in a breech or transverse position, which may necessitate medical intervention or special delivery techniques.

Immune System Enhancement: The baby's immune system receives antibodies from the mother, providing some protection against infections after birth.

Maturation of Organ Systems: The digestive and circulatory systems, along with other organ systems, continue to mature to support the baby's independent functioning.

Weight Gain: The baby gains a significant amount of weight during the third trimester, with the average weight gain being around half a pound per week.

Practice Breathing: The baby practices breathing movements, even though the lungs are not fully functional until birth.
As the due date approaches, the mother may experience various signs of impending labor, such as Braxton Hicks contractions, changes in the cervix, and the descent of the baby into the pelvic area.

Regular prenatal check-ups with healthcare providers help monitor the baby's growth and development, ensuring a healthy pregnancy and a smooth transition to labor and delivery. If you have specific concerns or questions about a pregnancy, it's always advisable to consult with a healthcare professional.

CHAPTER TWENTY-FIVE

CHILDBIRTH

Childbirth, also known as labor or parturition, is the process by which a baby is born from the mother's uterus. It typically occurs after a full-term pregnancy, which lasts about 40 weeks, but can vary. Childbirth is a complex physiological and emotional event that involves several stages:

1. Early Labor

Contractions Begin: The process often starts with mild contractions that gradually become more regular and intense.

Cervical Changes: The cervix begins to efface (thin out) and dilate (open) to allow the baby to pass through.

2. Active Labor

Increased Intensity: Contractions become stronger and closer together.

Cervical Dilation: The cervix continues to dilate, reaching around 10 centimeters to indicate full dilation.

Transition Phase: The final stage of active labor, marked by intense contractions as the baby moves into the birth canal.

3. Delivery

Pushing: The mother pushes during contractions, helping the baby move down the birth canal.

Birth of the Baby: The baby's head emerges first, followed by the rest of the body.

Umbilical Cord: This is the physical and emotional attachment between the mother and the fetus which should be clamped and cut.

4. Placental Stage

Delivery of the Placenta: The placenta, which provided nutrients to the baby, is expelled after the baby's birth.

Postpartum Period: The mother may continue to experience contractions as the uterus contracts to its pre-pregnancy size.

5. Postpartum Period

Recovery: The mother and baby are monitored for any complications. Bonding: Skin-to-skin contact and breastfeeding promote bonding.

Postpartum Care: Follow-up care for both the mother and the baby is essential.

Pain Management: Techniques such as epidurals or analgesics may be used to alleviate pain.

Monitoring: Fetal heart rate and maternal vital signs are closely monitored.

Cesarean Section: In some cases, a cesarean delivery may be performed if there are complications or medical indications.

CHAPTER TWENTY-SIX

WHO NAMES THE CHILD ?

The responsibility for naming a child typically falls on the child's parents or legal guardians. In many cultures and societies, it is customary for the parents to choose the name for their child. They may consider various factors, including cultural or family traditions, personal preferences, and the meaning or significance of the name.

In some cases, parents may also involve other family members or friends in the decision-making process or seek advice from religious or cultural leaders. Ultimately, the decision on a child's name is a personal one made by the parents or guardians, and the chosen name often reflects their values, beliefs, and cultural background.

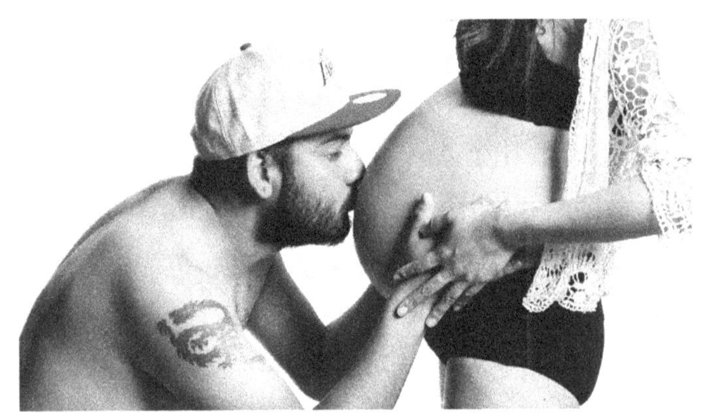

CHAPTER TWENTY-SEVEN

POSTPARTUM JOURNEY

The postpartum journey refers to the period of time following childbirth, typically lasting six weeks or longer, during which a woman's body undergoes physical and emotional changes as it transitions back to its pre-pregnancy state. This period is also commonly known as the postpartum or postnatal period.

Here are some key aspects of the postpartum journey:

Physical Recovery

Uterine Contractions: The uterus contracts to its pre-pregnancy size through a process called involution.

Vaginal Healing: If a woman has had a vaginal delivery, the perineum may need time to heal.

Cesarean Section Recovery: Women who undergo a cesarean section will have a longer recovery period as they heal from the surgical incision.

Hormonal Changes

Hormone Fluctuations: Hormone levels, especially estrogen and progesterone, undergo significant changes postpartum. This can contribute to mood swings and emotional adjustments.

Breast Changes: The body produces colostrum and then transitions to mature breast milk if the woman is breastfeeding.

Emotional Well-being:Baby Blues: Many women experience mood swings, tearfulness, and feelings of vulnerability in the first few days after childbirth. This is often referred to as "baby blues."

Postpartum Depression: Some women may experience more prolonged and severe mood disturbances, known as postpartum depression. It's essential to seek help if these symptoms persist.

Changes in Body Weight and Shape: Weight Loss: Some weight loss occurs naturally after childbirth due to the loss of amniotic fluid, placenta, and initial fluid retention.

Body Image: Women may have mixed feelings about their postpartum bodies. It's crucial to give the body time to recover and adjust.

Sleep Deprivation

Newborn Sleep Patterns: Infants typically have irregular sleep patterns, which can lead to sleep deprivation for new parents.

Fatigue: The demands of caring for a newborn can contribute to physical and mental fatigue.

Adjusting to Parenthood

Parental Roles: Both partners go through an adjustment period as they adapt to their new roles as parents.

Support System: A strong support system, including family, friends, and healthcare professionals, can be crucial during this time.

Postpartum Care

Follow-up Medical Care: Postpartum check-ups with healthcare providers are essential to monitor physical recovery and address any concerns.

Contraception: Discussions about family planning and contraception are often part of postpartum care.

Immediate Care:Ensure the baby's airways are clear, and they are breathing well.
Keep the baby warm and dry.
Administer eye ointment and a vitamin K shot, as recommended by healthcare professionals.

Apgar Score:Assess the baby's overall health using the Apgar score, which evaluates heart rate, breathing, muscle tone, reflexes, and color.

Umbilical Cord Care:Properly clamp and cut the umbilical cord as well as keeping it stump clean and dry to prevent any kind of infection.

Vaccinations:Administer vaccines as per the recommended schedule, often starting with the hepatitis B vaccine shortly after birth.

Newborn Screening:Conduct newborn screening tests to detect any potential health issues early on.

Mother-Baby Bonding:Encourage skin-to-skin contact between the baby and the mother to promote bonding.

Breastfeeding Support:Support and encourage breastfeeding, ensuring the baby latches properly.

Birth Registration:Complete necessary paperwork for the baby's birth certificate and registration.

Postpartum Care for Mother:Ensure the mother receives adequate postpartum care, including monitoring for any signs of complications.

Well-Baby Checkups:After putting to bed, always book regular well-baby checkups with a pediatrician to monitor growth and development of your baby.

Feeding and Nutrition:Establish a feeding schedule, whether breastfeeding or formula feeding, and introduce solid foods at the appropriate time.

Immunizations:Follow the recommended vaccination schedule to protect the child from various diseases.

Sleeping Arrangements:Create a safe sleeping environment, placing the baby on their back in a crib with no loose bedding.

Developmental Milestones:Monitor and celebrate developmental milestones, such as rolling over, sitting, crawling, and walking.

Parental Education and Support:Provide education and support for parents, including guidance on parenting techniques, safety measures, and recognizing signs of illness.

Dental Care:Introduce dental care, such as cleaning gums and teeth, as appropriate for the child's age.

Social Interaction:Encourage social interaction and play to support emotional and cognitive development.

Safety Measures:Baby-proof the home, keeping hazardous items out of reach and ensuring a safe environment.

Eye and Ear Checkups:Schedule regular checkups for eye and ear health.

Each child is unique, so it's essential to tailor care and interventions to their individual needs. Regular communication with healthcare professionals and staying informed about best practices in child development will contribute to a healthy and happy childhood.

The postpartum journey is unique to each woman, and the challenges and experiences can vary. Adequate support, both emotionally and physically, plays a vital role in ensuring a smooth transition into motherhood.

It's important for women to communicate openly with healthcare professionals, partners, and support networks to address any concerns and receive the necessary assistance during this transformative time.

It's important for women to communicate openly with healthcare professionals, partners, and support networks to address any concerns and receive the necessary assistance during this transformative time.

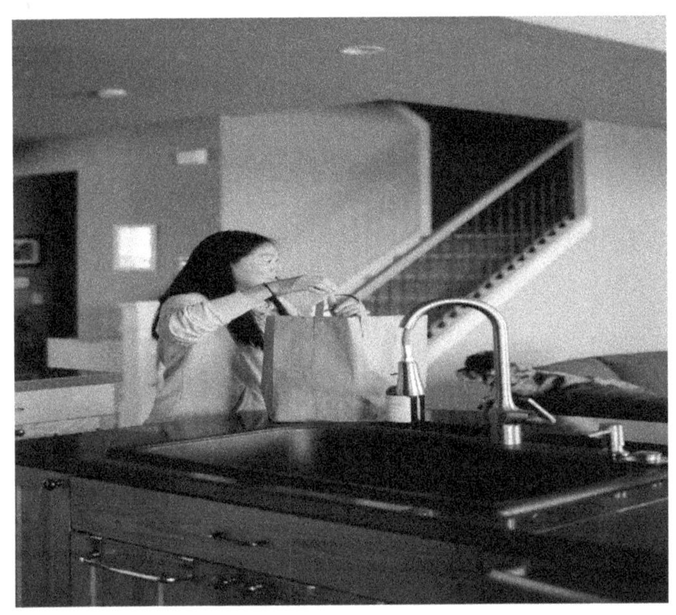

CHAPTER TWENTY-EIGHT

BATHING AN INFANT

Bathing a day-old baby requires special care and attention, as newborns are delicate and have sensitive skin. Here's a step-by-step guide on how to bathe a day-old baby:

1. Gather Supplies:Soft baby washcloths
Mild, fragrance-free baby soap
Lukewarm water
Soft baby towels
Diapers
Clean clothes
Cotton balls (optional)
Baby lotion (optional)

2. Choose the Right Time:Pick a time when both you and the baby are relaxed and not in a hurry.

3. Set the Room Temperature:Make sure the room is comfortably warm (around 75°F or 24°C) to prevent the baby from getting cold.

4. Wash Your Hands:Always wash your hands thoroughly before handling a newborn.

5. Prepare the Bathing Area: You can use a small baby bathtub or a clean sink for the first few weeks. Alternatively, you can use a soft towel or sponge to give a sponge bath.

7. Undress the Baby: Gently undress your baby, keeping them wrapped in a warm towel or blanket until you're ready to put them in the water.

8. Support the Baby's Head:
Always support the baby's head and neck with one hand while bathing and use your other hand to clean the baby's body.

9. Use Mild Soap Sparingly: Use a small amount of mild, fragrance-free baby soap on a soft washcloth or your hand. Gently wash the baby's body, starting with the face and moving down.

10. Pay Attention to Creases and Genital Area:Pay special attention to creases, such as behind the ears, under the arms, and in the neck folds. Use a soft cloth or cotton ball to clean the eyes, face, and genital area.

11. Rinse Thoroughly:Rinse your baby thoroughly with clean water. You can use a cup or your hand to pour water gently over the baby.

12. Pat Dry:Carefully lift your baby out of the water and pat them dry with a soft baby towel. Be gentle, especially in the creases.

13. Dress Your Baby:Dress your baby in clean, dry clothes, and don't forget to put on a diaper.

14. Apply Lotion (Optional):
If you choose to use baby lotion, apply a small amount to keep the baby's skin moisturized and ensure the lotion is suitable for newborns.

15. Enjoy the Bonding Time:Bathing can be a bonding experience, so talk to your baby and make the process as calm and soothing as possible.

Always be cautious, and if you have any concerns or questions about bathing your newborn, consult with your pediatrician for personalized advice.

CHAPTER TWENTY-NINE

CONCLUSION

Embarking on the exhilarating journey of fatherhood demands more than just anticipation—it requires active participation. As we delve into the comprehensive pregnancy guide for men, one crucial aspect stands out: the indispensable role of the expectant father. Antenatal care emerges as the compass guiding both partners through the intricate landscape of pregnancy.

These regular check-ups not only monitor the health of the mother but also provide invaluable insights into the development of the little one.

Navigating the trimesters of pregnancy becomes a shared experience, with each phase bringing new wonders and challenges. The expectant father's involvement is not merely a spectator sport; it's an active engagement in the symphony of life unfolding within the womb.

Understanding the physical and emotional changes of each trimester allows fathers to offer unwavering support, turning the journey into a collaborative adventure.

Amidst the excitement, maintaining optimal health is paramount. Fathers must prioritize their well-being, recognizing that a healthy partner begets a healthy pregnancy. Regular exercise, sufficient sleep, and stress management become allies in this shared endeavor. Simultaneously, embracing a wholesome diet ensures both partners are nourished, fostering a nurturing environment for the growing family.

In the culinary realm, "eating for two" takes on a new dimension. Choosing nutrient-rich foods and incorporating a variety of essential vitamins and minerals contributes not only to the well-being of the mother but also influences the baby's development. A balanced diet becomes a gesture of love, laying the foundation for a vibrant and resilient family.

As the curtains draw on this "Pregnancy Guide For Men", the spotlight is on the expectant father, whose active involvement shapes not just the journey but the destination—a thriving and harmonious family. Antenatal care, embracing the trimesters, staying healthy, and eating well are not mere checkpoints but the threads that weave the tapestry of a memorable and joyous pregnancy.

 So, gentlemen, let the adventure begin, hand in hand with the one you love, as you embark on the transformative odyssey of fatherhood.

Esteem Reader

I am taking a moment to express my sincere gratitude for choosing to explore the incredible world of fatherhood through our "Pregnancy Guide for Dads". Your decision to invest time in understanding and supporting your partner during this transformative journey speaks volumes about the amazing dad you're destined to be.

In the pages of this guide, I believe you saw a wealth of information, tips, and heartfelt advice to navigate the ups and downs of pregnancy with confidence and compassion. Your commitment to being an involved and supportive partner is not only commendable but also a testament to the love you have for both your partner and the little one on the way.

As you read through each chapter, you are not just learning about pregnancy; you actively participated in the beautiful tapestry of your growing family. Your willingness to engage in this process demonstrates your dedication to creating a nurturing and loving environment for your partner and the precious life developing within her.

The journey to parenthood is an awe-inspiring adventure filled with joy, challenges, and countless moments that will forever shape your family's story. Thank you for choosing to be an active participant in this incredible chapter of your life.

Wishing you wisdom, joy, and an abundance of love as you embrace the role of an extraordinary dad-to-be!

Warm regards,

Dora Harris

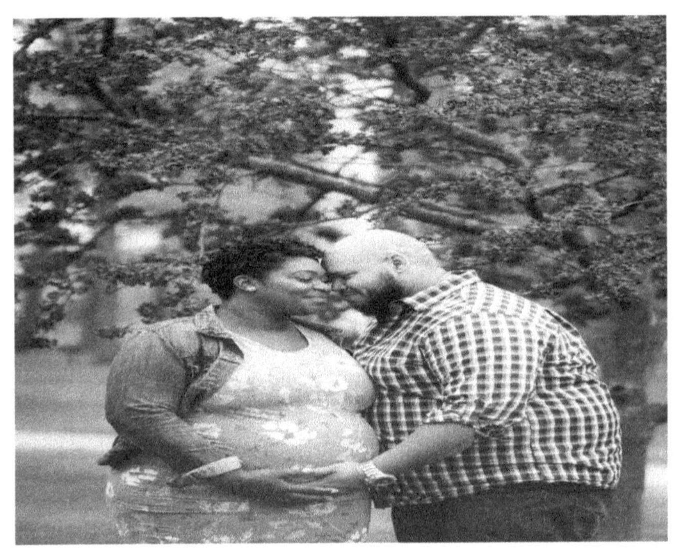